GUA SHA MANUAL
FOR NOVICES

ALL YOU NEED TO KNOW
ABOUT GUA SHA

ANDARA FARMER

Table of Contents

CHAPTER ONE

What you need to know about gua sha

Gua sha is a traditional East Asian healing technique. A lot of people use it to alleviate muscle pain and tension, but it's unclear how effective it is. We learn more about the efficacy and potential side effects of gua sha. Gua sha aims to circulate the body's energy, or qi or chi. A tool is used to rub the skin in long strokes, causing minor bruising in the process.

As scar tissue and connective tissues are broken down, joint mobility may be improved. Patients with certain medical conditions may not be able to benefit from the treatment.

What does gua sha mean?

Chinese medicine is the foundation of gua sha's practice (TCM). To be at your healthiest, TCM says your qi (pronounce "chi") must flow freely throughout your body. Stagnant qi, according to traditional Chinese medicine, can lead to health issues. It is common for acupuncturists to use a smooth-edged tool to gently scrape areas of the body where there is inflammation or stagnant qi in order to help improve circulation and promote healing through gua sha.

Most acupuncturists will use gua sha as a common treatment method." It can mean'scraping, rubbing, or pushing,' which is a reasonable translation. Sobo explains that "gua sha is basically just a tool-assisted type of massage.".

Differentiating Gua Sha Technique from the GASTON Technique

Muscle scraping can be used by physical therapists to help stretch and relax muscles and scar tissue. Gua sha-like techniques are referred to as Graston Techniques in the medical community. Amateur athlete David Graston brought gua sha to the United States in 1990. According to Sobo, the two methods of muscle scraping are nearly identical.

You can use the Graston Technique to perform gua sha

massage, but you can't trademark it. The main distinction is that Graston is administered by a physical therapist. They'll use anatomical or physiological terms to describe the procedure. As a result, you may hear more about promoting qi and blood circulation and breaking up the stagnation of energy in your body if you go to a very strict acupuncturist. But at the end of the day, both therapies aim for the same thing."

How often do acupuncturists use gua sha in their treatments?

Sobo points out that although acupuncturists are trained in gua sha, it isn't always offered during acupuncture sessions. It's possible that an acupuncturist has chosen not to perform this procedure because it doesn't make sense for the areas of the body being treated. However, if you'd like to try gua sha, you can always ask for it when you book your session.

CHAPTER TWO

Is gua sha bad for your health?

You might cringe at the mention of "scraping" in the context of gua sha. You won't be scrubbing your body like a windshield in the middle of winter with a practitioner's hands. As a general rule, gua sha is mild, but it can become more intense depending on the knots your acupuncturist finds.

This type of tool is known for its smooth and rounded edges. They won't hurt you in any way.

First, they'll apply a cream or lotion to the treatment area, and then adjust the intensity to your level of comfort. Acupuncturists don't just hammer a point in as hard as they can. Their goal is to break up these knots by locating the tense tissue, gently working on it, and gradually increasing the intensity until circulation is improved.

Uses

To alleviate muscle and joint pain, gua sha is most commonly used in China. Musculoskeletal disorders refer to conditions that affect the muscles and bones. Back pain, tendonitis, and carpal tunnel syndrome are a few examples.

Gua sha's proponents assert that it has anti-inflammatory and immune-boosting properties. Gua sha may be used to treat a cold, fever, or lung issues.

Microtrauma refers to minor injuries to the body, such as those caused by gua sha. These may help to break down scar tissue by causing a reaction in the body.

Fibrosis, a buildup of too much connective tissue as the body heals, may also benefit from microtrauma.

If the connective tissue isn't moving joints as it should, IASTM may be used by physiotherapists to help them. This may be a symptom of a more serious condition, like a repetitive strain injury. Other treatments, like stretching and strengthening exercises, can be used in conjunction with gua sha.

Benefits

On Pinterest, share

Gua sha may be beneficial to people who work at a computer and suffer from neck and shoulder pain, according to research.

In order to see if gua sha works, researchers have conducted small studies on the following groups:

Nearing menopause:

those who have neck and shoulder pain as a result of excessive computer usage

To aid in recovery after training for male weightlifters

seniors with back pain in old age

Many women reported an improvement in their perimenopausal symptoms after receiving gua sha.

Compared to a control group that received no treatment, gua

sha improved the range of motion and reduced pain in people who frequently used computers.

Weightlifters who had gua sha in 2017 reported that lifting heavier weights required less effort. This could imply that the therapy hastens muscle recovery.

Gua sha and a hot pack were used to treat back pain in older adults. Gua sha's effects lasted longer than those of other treatments, but both were effective.Trusted Source.

Gua sha patients experienced less back pain and more flexibility after just one week of treatment.

The dangers and side effects of taking medication.

Capillaries, which are small blood vessels near the skin's surface, are ruptured by gua sha. These bruises, referred to as sha, are typically red or purple in color.

In most cases, the bruises will heal in a few days or a week.

Pain and swelling can be eased by taking an over-the-counter analgesic like ibuprofen.

The bruised area should be protected and care should be taken to avoid bumping it. Inflammation and pain can both be relieved by using an ice pack.

While it is not recommended that gua sha practitioners break the skin during treatment, it is possible. Gua sha practitioners should sterilize their tools after each treatment to prevent the spread of infection.

Everyone isn't a good candidate for gua sha. Those who shouldn't receive gua sha include the following individuals:

• who are suffering from skin or vein disorders

• those who are prone to bleeding

• who are on blood thinner medication

• those with a history of deep vein thrombi

that hasn't completely healed from an infection, tumor, or previous wound

with a pacemaker or internal defibrillator implanted

Bodywork that uses gua sha

In order to get the best results, Sobo advises gua sha for the body to be tissue-dependent.

Gua sha is the best tool to use if you've got a knot in your muscles. To break up all of the adhesions, work perpendicular to the muscle fibers. Your muscles should be lengthened and aligned with their proper path once you've completed this step. With the knots in your upper shoulders, you'll want to use your tool to go back and forth across them. Your gua sha tool should be moved in the direction of the muscle fibers, which is usually inward to outward as you begin to loosen up. There are many reasons why you shouldn't begin gua sha in this direction.

CHAPTER THREE

For the face, use gua sha.

Those gua sha stones on faces have probably piqued your curiosity when you saw them on social media. In clinical studies, gua sha has been shown to decrease facial tension, puffiness, and inflammation, as well as sinus pressure. However, because the facial musculature is much thinner, you should exercise caution when working on this area.

"Unlike other muscles, the face's musculature is very thin and does not bulge up as much. Avoid dragging your tool from the outer edges of your face when using gua sha. Instead, divide your face into two halves and use your nose as the center. Work your way outward from your nose if you're doing it under your eyes with an outward-facing guasha tool. Maintain a straight path for your tool at all times. Don't slam your gua sha tool against your skin vigorously, as this will only cause the skin to become irritated and stretched. Keep things moving in a straight line, and apply pressure just enough to cause some redness but not enough to cause pain."

Before performing gua sha on your face, you can even use a lotion or serum to speed things up. Thus, the skin will be less likely to catch on your tool. Sobo recommends avoiding areas that are excessively swollen. Bruises can result from bursting capillary beds if you press too firmly into these.

Sobo recommends either a simple wooden spoon or a gemstone gua sha tool. No matter what you decide, make sure it's clean and in good working order.

It's impossible to tell the difference in terms of clinical efficacy." All you need is a tool that's simple to clean and keep in good working order. When something breaks or cracks, you don't want to use it any longer in case it chips or cracks. You don't want to rub your face with a jade gua sha face tool that has a small gash in it.

When working with a tool, Sobo advises using a clean one whenever possible. Boiling water or watered-down bleach solutions can be used to clean some tools, according to him.

Gua sha should be avoided by whom?

Gua sha is safe for the vast majority of people, but if you have circulation issues or diabetes, let your practitioner know before the session begins. Because of this, they'll be able to adjust the pressure to avoid any potential problems.

For someone with peripheral neuropathy, you might think gua sha would be too much, but Sobo says it isn't. Gua sha, when used in conjunction with acupuncture, can aid those with peripheral neuropathy in promoting blood flow. Gua sha, on the other hand, should be avoided or done with extreme caution if you're taking blood thinners.

As with most things, if you're uncomfortable, don't be afraid to speak up.

The intensity of acupuncture and gua sha can be a bit of a mystery if you've never had it done before. Know up front that you shouldn't feel any pain or discomfort as a result of these services. As soon as you notice that you're tensing up or digging your nails into the table, tell the practitioner right away so that they can make the necessary adjustments.

"The acupuncturist won't know if you don't say, 'Ouch, that hurts,' so get used to saying it. While this is going on, the acupuncturist should make it clear to you that the treatment won't help if you're in pain. They're attempting to de-stress the atmosphere. The acupuncturist will be running around in circles trying to make you feel better if the pain is too much for you to bear. This means that for you to find relief, everybody must be working together."

THE END

www.ingramcontent.com/pod-product-compliance
Lightning Source LLC
Chambersburg PA
CBHW050624160726

48003CB00003B/1321